Copyright © 2020 by Verona Jackson

RND

All rights reserved. No part of this
publication may be reproduced,
distributed, or transmitted in any form
or by any means, including
photocopying, recording, or other
electronic or mechanical methods,
without the prior written permission of
the publisher, except in the case of brief
quotations embodied in critical reviews
and certain other noncommercial uses
permitted by copyright law

Table of Contents

Introduction

Diabetes is a number of diseases that involve problems with the hormone insulin. Normally, the pancreas (an organ behind the stomach) releases insulin to help your body store and use the sugar and fat from the food you eat. Diabetes when one of the following occurs:

• When the pancreas does not produce any insulin.

• When the pancreas produces very little insulin.

• When the body does not respond appropriately to insulin, a condition called "insulin resistance."

Diabetes is a lifelong disease. Approximately 18.2 million Americans have the disease and almost one third (or approximately 5.2 million) are unaware that they have it. An additional 41 million people have prediabetes. As yet, there is no cure. People with diabetes need to manage their disease to stay healthy.

Without ongoing, careful management, diabetes can lead to a buildup of sugars in the blood, which can increase the risk of dangerous complications, including stroke and heart disease.

Different kinds of diabetes can occur, and managing the condition depends on the type. Not all forms of diabetes stem from a person being overweight or leading an inactive lifestyle. In fact, some are present from childhood.

The Role of Insulin in Diabetes

To understand why insulin is important, it helps to know more about how the body uses food for energy.

Your body is made up of millions of cells. To make energy, these cells need food in a very simple form. When you eat or drink, much of your food is broken down into a simple sugar called "glucose." Then, glucose is transported through the bloodstream to the cells of your body where it can be used to provide some of the energy your body needs for daily activities.

The amount of glucose in your bloodstream is tightly regulated by the hormone insulin. Insulin is always being released in small amounts by the pancreas. When the amount of glucose in your blood rises to a certain level, the pancreas will release more insulin to push more glucose into the cells. This causes the glucose levels in your blood (blood glucose levels) to drop.

To keep your blood glucose levels from getting too low (hypoglycemia or low blood sugar), your body signals you to eat and releases some glucose from the stores kept in the liver.

People with diabetes either don't make insulin or their body's cells no longer are able to recognize insulin, leading to high blood sugars. By definition, diabetes is having a blood glucose level of 126 milligrams per deciliter (mg/dL) or more after an overnight fast (not eating anything).

How insulin problems develop

Doctors do not know the exact causes of type 1 diabetes. Type 2 diabetes, also known as insulin resistance, has clearer causes.

Insulin allows the glucose from a person's food to access the cells in their body to supply energy. Insulin resistance is usually a result of the following cycle:

1. A person has genes or an environment that make it more likely that they are unable to make enough insulin to cover how much glucose they eat.

2. The body tries to make extra insulin to process the excess blood glucose.

3. The pancreas cannot keep up with the increased demands, and the excess blood sugar starts to circulate in the blood, causing damage.

4. Over time, insulin becomes less effective at introducing glucose to cells, and blood sugar levels continue to rise.

In the case of type 2 diabetes, insulin resistance takes place gradually. This is why doctors often recommend making lifestyle changes in an attempt to slow or reverse this cycle.

Types of Diabetes

Three major diabetes types can develop: Type 1, type 2, and gestational diabetes.

Type 1 diabetes:

Also known as juvenile diabetes, this type occurs when the body fails to produce insulin. People with type 1 diabetes are insulin-dependent, which means they must take artificial insulin daily to stay alive.

Type 2 diabetes:

Type 2 diabetes affects the way the body uses insulin. While the body still makes insulin, unlike in type I, the cells in the body do not respond to it as effectively as they once did. This is the most common type of diabetes, according to the National Institute of Diabetes and Digestive and Kidney Diseases, and it has strong links with obesity.

While most of these cases can be prevented, it remains for adults the leading cause of diabetes-related complications such as blindness, non-traumatic amputations and chronic kidney failure requiring dialysis. Type 2 diabetes usually occurs in people over age 40 who are overweight, but can occur in people who are not overweight. Sometimes referred to as "adult-onset diabetes," type 2 diabetes has started to appear more often in children because of the rise in obesity in young people.

Some people can manage their type 2 diabetes by controlling their weight, watching their diet, and exercising regularly. Others may also need to take a pill that helps their body use insulin better, or take insulin injections.

Often, doctors are able to detect the likelihood of type 2 diabetes before the condition actually occurs. Commonly referred to as pre-diabetes, this condition occurs when a person's blood glucose levels are higher than normal, but not high enough for a diagnosis of type 2 diabetes.

Gestational diabetes:

This type occurs in women during pregnancy when the body can become less sensitive to insulin. Gestational diabetes does not occur in all women. The condition occurs in approximately 4% of all pregnancies and usually resolves after giving birth.

Pregnant women who have an increased risk of developing gestational diabetes are those who are over 25 years old, are above their normal body weight before pregnancy, have a family history of diabetes or are Hispanic, black, Native American, or Asian.

Screening for gestational diabetes is performed during pregnancy. Left untreated, gestational diabetes increases the risk of complications to both the mother and her unborn child.

Usually, blood glucose levels return to normal within six weeks of childbirth. However, women who have had gestational diabetes have an increased risk of developing type 2 diabetes later-in-life.

Prediabetes

Doctors refer to some people as having prediabetes or borderline diabetes when blood sugar is usually in the range of 100 to 125 milligrams per deciliter (mg/dL).

Normal blood sugar levels sit between 70 and 99 mg/dL, whereas a person with diabetes will have a fasting blood sugar higher than 126 mg/dL.

The prediabetes level means that blood glucose is higher than usual but not so high as to constitute diabetes.

People with prediabetes are, however, at risk of developing type 2 diabetes, although they do not usually experience the symptoms of full diabetes.

The risk factors for prediabetes and type 2 diabetes are similar. They include:

- being overweight

- a family history of diabetes

- having a high-density lipoprotein (HDL) cholesterol level lower than 40 mg/dL or 50 mg/dL

- a history of high blood pressure

- having gestational diabetes or giving birth to a child with a birth weight of more than 9 pounds

- a history of polycystic ovary syndrome (PCOS)

- being of African-American, Native American, Latin American, or Asian-Pacific Islander descent

- being more than 45 years of age

- having a sedentary lifestyle

If a doctor identifies that a person has prediabetes, they will recommend that the individual makes healthful changes that can ideally stop the progression to type 2 diabetes. Losing weight and having a more healthful diet can often help prevent the disease.

What Are the Symptoms of Type 1 Diabetes

The symptoms of type 1 diabetes often occur suddenly and can be severe. They include:

• Increased thirst.

• Increased hunger (especially after eating).

• Dry mouth.

• Frequent urination.

• Unexplained weight loss (even though you are eating and feel hungry).

• Fatigue (weak, tired feeling).

• Blurred vision.

• Labored, heavy breathing (Kussmaul respirations).

• Loss of consciousness (rare).

What Are the Symptoms of Type 2 Diabetes

The symptoms of type 2 diabetes may be the same as those listed above. Most often, there are no symptoms or a very gradual development of the above symptoms. Other symptoms may include:

- Slow-healing sores or cuts.

- Itching of the skin (usually in the vaginal or groin area).

- Yeast infections.

- Recent weight gain.

- Numbness or tingling of the hands and feet.

- Impotence or erectile dysfunction.

General Symptoms of Diabetes In The Body.

- Being more thirsty than usual

- Passing more urine

- Feeling tired

- Always feeling hungry

- Having cuts that heal slowly

- Itching, skin infections

- Blurred vision

- Unexplained weight loss (type 1)

- Gradually putting on weight (type 2)

- Headaches

- Feeling dizzy

- Leg cramps.

Diabetes Complications

High blood sugar damages organs and tissues throughout your body. The higher your blood sugar is and the longer you live with it, the greater your risk for complications.

Complications associated with diabetes include:

- heart disease, heart attack, and stroke

- neuropathy

- nephropathy

- retinopathy and vision loss

- hearing loss

- foot damage such as infections and sores that don't heal

- skin conditions such as bacterial and fungal infections

- depression

- dementia

Diabetes Diagnosis

Anyone who has symptoms of diabetes or is at risk for the disease should be tested. Women are routinely tested for gestational diabetes during their second or third trimesters of pregnancy.

Doctors use these blood tests to diagnose prediabetes and diabetes:

- The fasting plasma glucose (FPG) test measures your blood sugar after you've fasted for 8 hours.

- The A1C test provides a snapshot of your blood sugar levels over the previous 3 months.

- To diagnose gestational diabetes, your doctor will test your blood sugar levels between the 24th and 28th weeks of your pregnancy.

- During the glucose challenge test, your blood sugar is checked an hour after you drink a sugary liquid.

- During the 3 hour glucose tolerance test, your blood sugar is checked after you fast overnight and then drink a sugary liquid.

- The earlier you get diagnosed with diabetes, the sooner you can start treatment. Find out whether you should get tested, and get more information on tests your doctor might perform.

Diabetes Prevention

Type 1 diabetes isn't preventable because it's caused by a problem with the immune system. Some causes of type 2 diabetes, such as your genes or age, aren't under your control either.

Yet many other diabetes risk factors are controllable. Most diabetes prevention strategies involve making simple adjustments to your diet and fitness routine.

If you've been diagnosed with prediabetes, here are a few things you can do to delay or prevent type 2 diabetes:

• Get at least 150 minutes per week of aerobic exercise, such as walking or cycling.

• Cut saturated and trans fats, along with refined carbohydrates, out of your diet.

• Eat more fruits, vegetables, and whole grains.

• Eat smaller portions.

• Try to lose 7 percentTrusted Source of your body weight if you're overweight or obese.

Treatment for Diabetes (Insulin Plant)

Spiral flag or insulin plant, as it is commonly known in India, is a perennial plant. Its scientific name is Costus igneus, and it belongs to the family Costaceae. The herbal plant is upright with beautiful flowers. It has spiral leaves from where it derives its name.

Multiple studies have shown that this plant contains anti-diabetic properties. It has its origins from Central and South America. In Southern parts of India, it is grown as an ornamental plant. For ages, it has been widely used as an Ayurvedic treatment for diabetes mellitus in India. It is used as a natural remedy for renal diseases in Mexico.

Components of the Plant

The spiral flag is rich in antioxidants such as ascorbic acid, a-tocopherol, b-carotene, steroids and flavonoids. It also contains large amounts of proteins, triterpenoids, iron, alkaloids, and carbohydrates.

How is this Plant Ingested

There are two ways in which the leaves of the plant are ingested to relieve the symptoms of diabetes.

Fresh leaves are crushed, and the juice is taken orally. Another way is to chew it directly. The recommended dose is two leaves in the morning at the beginning of the herbal treatment. After a week, it is gradually reduced to one leaf in the morning and evening. Leaves are dried in the shade. After that, they are crushed and powdered. The powder is taken orally mixed with water. The recommended dosage for an adult is one teaspoon per day.

Why is it Effective in the Treatment of Diabetes

The primary reason why the insulin plant is effective in arresting the symptoms of diabetes is the presence of phyto-compounds. This component is also referred to as natural insulin. The phyto-compounds in conjunction with the other properties of the plant mimic the metabolic activity of insulin. It is particularly effective when ingested inside the body.

The green leaves also contain corosolic acid which enhances the production of insulin in the body. Increased insulin in the body keeps hyperglycemia in check.

It lowers blood sugar levels in diabetic patients, especially those with type-2 diabetes. The plant extracts produce sensitivity of the pancreas, and it increases the production of insulin in the blood.

It is also shown to reduce the glucose levels in the blood. In many studies, it has also demonstrated a considerable decrease in the level of cholesterol as well as triglycerides in the body. This hypolipidemic activity is most effective against the fats and cholesterol that is induced by diabetes.

Apart from diabetic benefits, the plant possesses anti-inflammatory, anti-cancer and anti-microbial properties. The liquid extracts also cause increased production of potassium and sodium which has a significant effect on dieresis.

Precautionary Measures

Although the plant extracts are not associated with toxicity or side effects, it is not the best treatment for diabetic patients who have a history of coronary ailments. Pregnant women or someone nursing a baby should not ingest the extracts of the insulin plant.

How To Make Insulin Leaves Extract

Directions:

- Select a bunch of insulin leaves (10-15) and wash it under flowing water.
- Cut the leaves into small pieces and dry them under the sun.

- You can check the drying of the leaves by squeezing it.

- Once the leaves are dried, store it in an airtight jar.

- Take a cup of water and boil it.

- Once it is boiled, pour the water into a glass containing the dried insulin plant leaves.

- Wait until the water turns brown.

- Drink the extract on regular basis for positive results.

Healthy Recipe Insulin Tea

Ingredients

- 5-7 insulin leaves

- 4 cups of water

*   Honey for taste

Directions

*   Wash the leaves and let it dry out.

*   Boil the water in a pot.

*   As the water begins to boil, add the leaves.

*   Let it boil, till the water reduces to one cup.

*   Filter the tea and pout the tea into a cup.

*   Add honey for taste.

Side Effects of Insulin Plant

As usual, every herb that holds a plethora of benefits

is bound to have some risks incorporated with it. In the

case of insulin plant, it is no different.

- Pregnant and lactating women must avoid it, as the herb may affect the hormonal balance.

- Avoid consuming the leaves directly because of the strong taste and effect can cause a burning sensation.

Health Benefits Of Insulin Plant

From normalising the blood sugar levels to improving digestion, the advantages of the herb are limitless.

1. Cures Diabetes

The herb works wonders by reducing the high sugar level in your blood. The fructose content in the insulin leaves regulate the sugar levels, by maintaining it in the required level. Regular consumption of the leaves can aid in preventing the onset of chronic health complications developed as a result of diabetes. Such as the uncontrolled flow of nutrients in the body as well as organ failures. A decoction made out of the leaves is the best cure for diabetes.

2. Improves Digestion

The various complex components, vitamins and nutrients present in the herb are asserted to work similar to the E.coli bacteria, which improves the digestion process. By acting as a natural pre-biotic, it actuates smooth digestion. The growth of the good bacteria in the digestive system aids in the proper absorption of nutrients. Likewise, the fructose level helps to improve the colon function, easing the excretion process.

3. Possesses Antioxidant Properties

Studies have revealed that the insulin plant has compounds that are antioxidative in nature. The antioxidative property of the herb destroys the free radicals, thereby protecting your body and cells. The antioxidant properties of the herb are concentrated in the methanolic extracts found in the rhizomes and leaves of the plant.

4. Manages Diuresis

The herb possesses sodium and water retention capacity, making it an integral part of improving your bladder and kidney health. The rhizomes and leaves of the plant have diuretic property and manage diuresis.

5. Has Antibacterial Properties

The methanolic extract from the plant protects your body from gram-positive species like Bacillus megaterium, Bacillus cerus, Staphylococcus aureus and various gram-negative strains like Escherichia coli, Pseudomonas aeruginosa, Klebsiella pneumoniae, and Salmonella typhimurium. It kills the problem causing bacteria and provides relief in the excretory process.

6. Cures Liver Problems

Insulin plant helps break down the fat deposits and unnecessary toxins in the liver. By removing the toxins from your body, the herb limits the development of chronic illnesses in the future. Breaking down of the fatty acids help in improving the liver function as well.

Regular consumption of the herb is an effective solution for curing liver problems.

7. Improves Bladder Health

Being diuretic in nature, the insulin plant is effective in curing problems related to the bladder system. Regular consumption of the herb can aid in stimulating the proper functioning of your bladder, avoiding the risks of developing any infections.

8. Enhances Immunity

The antioxidant properties of the herb are effective in improving your immune system. Insulin plant removes the toxins such as free radicals and helps develop a healthy immune system. Regular consumption can improve the immune system and shield your body from any illness.

9. Prevents Cancer

Studies have revealed that the insulin plant has antiproliferative and anticancer properties. Along with its antioxidant nature, the herb helps by removing the free radicals that cause cancer. It was ascertained that the herb is exclusively useful in treating the HT 29 and A549 cells. Regular consumption of the herb helps prevent the growth of cancerous cells in our body.

10. Reduces Cholesterol Levels

The insulin herb is rich in water-soluble components that aid in slowing down the absorption of glucose into the blood system. By slowing down the process, it regulates the sugar absorption and insulin production in the body. The slow absorption results in the proper absorption of the fat content and hence, resulting in the reduction of blood cholesterol levels. Thereby, the herb helps your body from succumbing to the risks of heart attack, stroke, or cancer.

11. Treats Sore Throat

One of the other features of the miracle herb is its anti-inflammatory properties. Consuming the herb can help cure a sore throat and symptoms of bronchitis as it is developed due to the inflammation of your airways. Insulin plant will reduce the inflammation and cure the condition.

12. Reduces Blood Pressure

Insulin herb is known to subside hypertension. Regular consumption of the herb will aid in reducing high levels of blood pressure and calming the heart.

13. Cures Asthma

As mentioned before, the plant has anti-inflammatory properties that aid in clearing any inflammation caused in the airways. It helps cure asthma by soothing the lung muscles that tighten on the onset of an asthma attack.

Dosage Of Insulin Plant

Singularly dependent on the individual's physical condition, the dosage is not exactly specified. However, in order to gain the health benefits offered by the herb, it is recommended that it be consumed at least twice per day. Consuming it more than twice have not resulted in any side effects, but consult a physician if you want to increase your dosage.

You can consume it once in the morning and once before going to bed at night. Insulin plant can be used as a potion (leaves extract), or insulin leaves tea can be made to enjoy its health benefits.

Care instructions for insulin plant

Propagation of insulin plant– Insulin plant can be propagated both by root and stem cuttings. Ensure that the rhizome contains at least 3-4 leaves, before separating the plant from the mother plant. Try to choose a place with partial sun or partial shade and dig the soil about an inch or two and plant the rhizome. The same condition applies when you are planting with stem cuttings; ensure that the stem cuttings are about 3-4 inches in length.

Soil conditions:

The insulin plant requires well-aerated and well-drained soil. It does not grow well in salty and sandy soil; however, the plant likes compost soil.

Temperature –The plant likes warm temperatures and love to grow at 35 to 45 degrees of temperature.

Water:

The insulin plant loves moisture and plenty of water, always ensure that the soil is wet, and water the plants more often. Ensure that the soil is not water-logged.

Sunlight:

Protect your insulin plant from direct sunlight. The insulin plant requires partial sunlight to produce healthy leaves. Also, avoid putting your insulin plant in complete shade. If you are planting it indoors ensure that the plant gets enough light.